INVISIBLE
INK

How to Become Your Most Excellent

P. SPENCER

BALBOA.
PRESS
A DIVISION OF HAY HOUSE

Balboa Press books may be ordered through booksellers or by contacting:

Balboa Press
A Division of Hay House
1663 Liberty Drive
Bloomington, IN 47403
www.balboapress.com
1 (877) 407-4847

Because of the dynamic nature of the Internet, any web addresses or links contained in this book may have changed since publication and may no longer be valid. The views expressed in this work are solely those of the author and do not necessarily reflect the views of the publisher, and the publisher hereby disclaims any responsibility for them.

The author of this book does not dispense medical advice or prescribe the use of any technique as a form of treatment for physical, emotional, or medical problems without the advice of a physician, either directly or indirectly. The intent of the author is only to offer information of a general nature to help you in your quest for emotional and spiritual well-being. In the event you use any of the information in this book for yourself, which is your constitutional right, the author and the publisher assume no responsibility for your actions.

Any people depicted in stock imagery provided by Thinkstock are models, and such images are being used for illustrative purposes only.
Certain stock imagery © Thinkstock.

Print information available on the last page.

ISBN: 978-1-5043-4853-9 (sc)
ISBN: 978-1-5043-4854-6 (e)

Library of Congress Control Number: 2015921445

Balboa Press rev. date: 12/31/2015

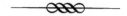

To my beautiful daughter, Lauren.

Your unconditional love, wisdom, and
laughter are my infinite inspiration.

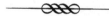

Frame Your Brain: The Precept

The mind is everything; what you think you become.

—Buddha

My mission is to be your catalyst in reaching the best you can be. As a nurse practitioner with years of experience in the health care arena, I want to share with you the invaluable power of the human mind and its ability to attain the outcomes and dreams you desire. Throughout my career, I have had the privilege to witness how powerful the human mind is and the invisible force it has to rise above any storm. This has had an immense impact in my life and has struck something deep within me. We all have the capacity and power to govern our own lives. Because I have personally seen countless miracles occur in the lives of many, my wish for you is that amazing miracles will come into your life.

As we all know, life is not easy. Challenges and difficulties come, often without warning. But what if through these life challenges we could elevate ourselves to become stronger, more fulfilled, and happier individuals? This is a significant question many of my patients, their families, and I face when a major shift occurs. We cannot change the past difficulties we have endured, but we can reframe the experiences in our minds as to how we accept them. As for the title of this book, the word invisible is the intangible of our mind power and the word ink refers to our experiences that cannot be erased.

What does it take to go beyond the invisible limits that our minds try to confine us to? One of the important elements we need to be open to is when we take the time and effort to believe in ourselves and a higher power, the impossible can be created. In working with patients, families, and many individuals, I have learned that the pathway to reaching our highest selves lies in the power of our minds. When I am asked how people with incredible challenges, various diseases, physical or emotional limitations, or significant loss overcome these challenges, the answer is that this power lies in all of us, in our minds and in our wills.

You are the artist, the architect who creates what you so desire. We are each given the freedom to design the pictures of our life. And just as everyone is unique and distinct, so are the creative opportunities before us. Following higher thinking, positive attitudes and actions, affirmations, and the intuition you and I are born with is key to attaining excellence. Every one of us has a genius inside. We all need to embrace our imprinted desires, passions, and strengths of mind, for they can assist us in producing the lives we choose to live. Achieving this takes truly knowing ourselves and knowing that there is an inner, intangible light that connects us to our life experiences. Trusting in ourselves enables us each to design the most beautiful blueprint of which each of us is meant to be. This occurs by framing our minds with positive thinking and meditation and using the power that awaits us to create unlimited boundaries.

If you could design the life you have always wanted, what would it look like? If you took a photograph of it, what would you see? How would it feel? Time is an invisible bridge, and you should not let it place limits in life. Let it elevate you to the majestic and most powerful person you are meant to be.

We each create our own destiny through our thoughts, actions, and the environment we put ourselves in. This affects emotional, mental, physical, and spiritual health. One of my favorite quotes from Gandhi is, "Set in motion this self-controlled power with your attitude, which additionally can cause boundless victory in your life." When faced with struggles in life, no matter how big or small, our thoughts and attitudes direct our way. Inner wisdom, strength, and higher thinking lead us to having stronger and enlarged selves. How can we reach higher thinking even in the face of struggles? We all are born with an internal power that is invisible. It is spiritual wisdom.

Without a doubt, we can all think of life experiences that have challenged us. Whether big or small, they often occur without warning, catching us by surprise and many times in disbelief. All human beings have to deal with these things. As for me, my most profound and explosive life-changing experience occurred approximately eight years ago, when I suddenly and unexpectedly lost my husband in a snowmobiling accident. Life as I knew it was forever changed. I never thought I would be raising a child alone, let alone being faced with so many adversities along the way. How was I going to forge through this extremely deep and treacherous storm?

At the same time of this immense crisis, other challenges engulfed me perilously. Two family members who were diagnosed with Huntington's disease, a disease that does not yet have a cure, fought and lost their long fights. With heartfelt sadness, I had questions that remained unanswered, yet I felt I needed to move forward in all aspects of my life. I did so, of course, with fortitude and determination. In retrospect, I have been transmuted in so many ways.

We know how precious and fragile life can be. It is with faith and steadfast hope that we can choose to elevate ourselves to be stronger and more determined individuals through our experiences. No matter where you and I are in this life, adversities can jolt us, but with strength and life choices we all can overcome profound changes in our lives. I believe in you and the possibility to overcome challenges and adversities. I believe you can move from worry, doubt, and fear to a life of transformation, just as my patients and I have done. When you are at the crossroads of life, know that the answers are within you and that an inner light leads the way. The pivotal points in my life have given me immense courage, strength, determination, and happiness, and I want you to experience this too. You are a winner— no matter what you are dealing with. Gaining a deeper understanding in the power of love, forgiveness, and in having faith that there is a higher source, continues to lead me to success and in fulfilling my dreams. This is my infrastructure for life.

In the quietness of my heart, I know this inner light is very powerful and invisibly directs the design of my life, as it does yours. What led me into a heartfelt nursing career was when, at the age of seventeen, I stood in awe of how angelic the nurses caring for my grandfather were. That day I knew my life's work would be to care for patients; I knew nursing was a calling I was meant to follow. I continue to feel privileged to care for others and provide comfort and hope in their times of need.

I am sure you can think of a family member, a friend, or someone that has impacted your life, and changed you or your circumstances in some way. This change may have come from a painful experience or one involving deep emotional connections. The challenges and adversities we all face can also provide us with unforeseen opportunities. As for me, the significant loss of my grandfather and other family members has left an imprint on my soul that pushes me above and beyond what I thought I could accomplish in my life and in helping others. This imprinted mark on my soul continues to give my life purpose and to allow me the opportunity to help others in various ways. Life is challenging; that we all know. It is with fortitude and willpower that we grow stronger and that we design our dreams. The quiet voice within all of us directs our lives into happiness, fulfillment, and other positive outcomes. It is in the silence of our days that we can become in tune with our higher thinking and knowing. This tuning in to the quiet voice within has been called intuition, instinct, or a higher power of knowing. No matter what the term, it is this flow of knowing that governs us as human beings.

How you have handled challenges and adversities in the past and where they have brought you thus far are both significant with regard to the next set of decisions you will make. We all face challenges and setbacks, but the courses we travel and the life paths we choose are what define our futures. Though you may find yourself struggling with these, no matter how big or small, perseverance opens the door for us and enable us recover and move forward.

Have you excelled in self-growth through these trials, or have they held you back? *Adversity Advantage,* a book written by Dr. Paul Stoltz and Eric Weihenmayer, is extremely insightful. It has given me the opportunity to be a conduit for the patients I care for, who also face adversities. In this book, Dr. Stoltz discusses how adversity can affect each of us: "When it comes to adversity, the most important issues are not whether you are in complete control. What matters most is how much influence you believe you have in any given situation."

Eric Weihenmayer, Dr. Stoltz's cowriter, has written about overcoming physical challenges and finding his own greatness after losing his eyesight in ninth grade. He has climbed seven mountains around the world without sight. He is a remarkable example of how to handle adversity. He says, "I believe that inside each of us is something I can only describe as a light, which has the capacity to feed on adversity, to consume it like fuel. When we tap into that light, every frustration, every setback, every obstacle becomes a brighter source to power. The greater the challenge, the brighter the light burns. Through it, we become more focused; more creative, more driven, and can even learn to transcend our own perceived limitations to bring our lives more meaning." Without a doubt, we can all think of situations that have confronted us with difficulty. Assessing how you have responded to them in the past is very important. Have these trials or adversities held you back, or have they helped you emerge to a better and stronger you?

In being able to help so many patients, their families, and others who have given me the opportunity to care for them as a nurse practitioner, I have continually witnessed the power of the mind and all it can accomplish. Their accomplishments and journeys have resulted from their choices and from their openness to change. We all must realize the power that doubt and fear have in our life can hold us back if we choose to let them. When you ask yourself important questions as to what you find yourself thinking about, what is it that you give your focus of attention to in your life are important questions to answer for yourself. Is your process of thinking causing stress, doubt, anxiety, or fear in you? If the answer is yes, then this type of mental battlement is limiting you from your life's happiness, peace, joy, and the dreams you wish to fulfill. Our minds influence our self- belief and instead of allowing our minds to cause thoughts that produce suffocating and unwanted outcomes, make the choice to allow your thinking pattern one of positive and thinking. This can be overcome by changing mental stagnation and negative thinking to a dynamic state of peace, gratitude, and joy. Use your mental power as a conduit for success. Otherwise, negative thoughts can gain an invisible control that limits all of life's enrichment and happiness—and these are yours to claim. Feeling that you have lost control can lead to anxiety, frustration, and mental fatigue. This can allow you to feel defeated, a feeling that needs to be overcome. When you feel defeated, the influence of this negative power wins. You can, however, regain control by resonating positive changes and outcomes through your power of thoughts.

Therefore, the blueprint starts with you and your thinking. The key for each and every one of us starts with the power of our minds, which is limitless. This knowledge is significant to how we bridge success, happiness, peace, and contentment. Deliberate and positive thinking begins with developing and enlarging the foundation upon which you can build the person you wish to be. When we stretch our thinking, we need to open our minds to all that is possible and realize the invisible power of our thoughts are what truly directs our lives. Therefore, our achievements and human happiness we so desire are waiting for us through the power of our minds. When you and I experience happiness and fulfillment, the energy it produces is very powerful.

Over the years I have read and studied the power of higher thinking through the writings of many well-known authors, including Ernest Holmes, who was a great teacher, lecturer, and writer. He has given great insight into the power of the mind and all that it can accomplish. His book, *Living the Science of Mind*, has invaluable teachings for living life fully by changing our thinking. He has written about the magnitude of power that the law of attraction has. This is something you may or may not think about in great detail, but I would like to share with you the phenomenon of the law of attraction and all that it can conquer. Ernest Holmes, through his writings and teachings, which came into being as early as 1915, has given many individuals over the years the gift of insight into how thinking affirmatively can have great impact and power in our lives. His teachings continue to resonate today.

Holmes identifies the power of affirmative thinking in three ways. First, it is important to realize that "we are surrounded by a Creative Mind which reacts to our thoughts. This is the basis of all faith and all effective prayer." Have you ever considered just how powerful our thoughts are in our lives? Our minds are always active, whether we are conscious of it or not. Negative thoughts influence us differently than positive thoughts. Choosing to have positive thoughts creates the power of attracting positive influences in our lives. Therefore, "let us begin with the thought that we are all united with an Invisible Force which is creative, and that we are already one with a Universal Mind which can do anything."

Second, Holmes explains that our minds are actively thinking centers and that the sum total of our thoughts is either silently attracting goodness or repelling it from us. As he and others have taught, about 90 percent of our thinking is unconscious. When we are about to fall sleep at night, our last conscious thoughts hold the power to influence the thoughts our subconscious minds work through during the hours we sleep each night.

These thoughts then set in motion that which our conscious mind thinks about in the morning upon waking. This is the invisible and influential bridge between states of consciousness; it is imperative to pay close attention to your thoughts and the power of their influence as they move across this unconscious bridge.

Third, Holmes teaches that "we can change our thinking and in so doing cause the law of mind to act affirmatively for us instead of negatively." He also says, "The affirmative attitude will always overcome the negative." Individually, we control our own thoughts and, in becoming aware of this throughout the day, can produce positive effects. One of the affirmations he has taught includes saying this every day and believing it: "I do accept this good. I do believe my prayer is answered. I do affirm the presence of love, friendship, prosperity, health, and peace or whatever the need may be-and nothing in me denies, rejects, or refutes it. I do accept it." Our thoughts and attitudes should be used to produce supreme good in our lives and in the lives of others. This is something we each can control. Practicing daily positive affirmations can bring positive changes to our lives that will create expansive new realities for each and every one of us.

As we are well aware, the external world attempts to influence our thinking by the reflection on what the world's current ideas, trends or beliefs are and that they should also be ours. Outside influences and comparisons with others additionally attempts to diminish our self-worth. It takes acknowledgement and self-awareness to not allow the pressures of social and cultural norms dictate who you are. Additionally, consumerism can also have a negative influence on our thinking patterns. Therefore we all need to protect our minds and the power that external influences attempts to place on us. *Stretch your thinking* and believe in yourself. We are all unique individuals with special gifts and talents. Love yourself and celebrate you who. You and I were each created with a unique design. Be kind to yourself and listen to the loving voice of truth within you.

You and I were born with love and all the inner guidance that we need. As infants and children, our internal design directed us to eat when we were hungry and to meet all the basic needs we required for optimal growth. It was love, kindness, a gentle spirit, and an inner knowing that guided us in harmony. Yet as we grow up and are exposed to all the external influences society attempts to conform us to, we seem to lose our sense of self, self-worth, and self-love. This external noise can have the power to cause self-doubt and a sense of inadequacy. Imbalance happens, and we start telling ourselves false messages. You and I are to love ourselves as we have been created to do. We must be mindful of this throughout our days and trust ourselves and the gentle voice within us as we did when we were young. We need to commit to ourselves consciously to be open to all life has to offer us in peace, harmony, and balance.

In some ways, as Ernest Holmes indicates, we should permit our consciousness to range in the field of greater possibilities. And to accomplish this, he states, "A certain time should be taken each day for the enlargement of consciousness. This is done by reminding our imagination that the field with which it deals is limitless, that Mind is the Creator and Sustainer, the Mind is Infinite, ever available, and always responsive to us." You have an inner voice of wisdom that quietly leads you to wanting to become a more fulfilled and happy individual. Accomplishing this involves trusting yourself to being open to it. And even though the trials of life challenge us, ultimately they should propel us to be stronger, more confident, and happier individuals. Knowing this and listening to your inner voice is your bridge to a more fulfilled life. A powerful force available to us is meditation. When the mind is focused on love and positive affirmations, negative thought patterns dissipate, and the flow of positive energy and direction is able to enter. Think about the positive things you want in life and picture them over and over again every day. Resonant and intertwine your thoughts with the emotions of already having what your heart so desires as if you have already received that which you wish for. It is additionally important to also speak your positive affirmations out loud, as this energy is very powerful. Verbalizing positive statements of that which you think radiates positive energy into the universe and this positive energy flows back to us. This is called the law of attraction and this is what Ernest Holmes spoke about.

I am sure many of us have had doubts and fears in our life journeys, but there comes a time when the power of fear should not hold us back from becoming who we truly want to be. Fear is an invisible chain that constrains us. Breaking fearful thought patterns and gaining positive control in our mind is vital to unlocking this invisible chain. With daily positive thinking and meditation and by reaffirming to ourselves, "I am strong, I am fearless, I am peace, I am love, and I am beautifully designed with my inner light leading my way," we harness the invisible power within. This can produce a new reality in our life.

As for the challenges in my life and in my patients' lives, all of which involve overcoming doubt and fear, I teach that we need to believe with our minds and hearts in the power within us to lead balanced and fulfilled lives. I have changed the meaning of the word *fear* by breaking down its letters into *favor, energy, abundance,* and *reignite.* Believe in and expect great *favor* in life, as your thoughts have the power to create positive actions. Controlling thinking patterns with positive words and thoughts negates the power of the negative. This allows the mind to produce positive *energy* that flows from us.

As you know and as the laws of physics teach, energy is power. The world of science continues to expand in many arenas of study, including the study of human energy and the energy that surrounds us. Scientific inquiry over many years has brought into place an acknowledgement that the "body" of the human being does not end with the skin. It is a scientific fact that human beings have an electromagnetic field and energy centers, also called the "subtle body," that extends beyond the skin. Studies in various disciplines have come to their own individual conclusions about how to verify the bio-field (Brennan, 1993). Many of these documented studies can be found in physics, biology, chemistry, and engineering, among other disciplines. In a book called *Light Energy, The Journey of Personal Healing* by B. Brennan explains that energy is present in nature, in the objects we live with, in the food we eat, in the sounds we hear, in the colors we are exposed to, in the fragrances we smell, in the exercising we do, and in the human body in general. Therefore, being aware of all of these play an intricate role in life, in addition to what the mind attracts to us. It is vital when making conscious decisions to replace negative thoughts that impede our positive energy flow. Negative thoughts produce negative energy, but choosing positive thoughts can create positive energy. Positive thoughts create healthy energy and greatly influence our life. I am sure many of you have heard the saying "like attracts like." Why not attract positive things into your life? Attracting the positive can range from peace, joy, happiness, contentment, health, friendship, and abundance to a world full of infinite beautiful possibilities.

Abundance is the blueprint for what life should look like, and your inner voice is waiting to be heard and to guide you. You and I need to pay attention to it. *Reignite* your inner spark. A higher plane of reality connects us to that which is unseen but felt deep within. Each and every one of us have the ability to shine with brilliant color and to experience immense love, joy, happiness, contentment, and success if we allow our minds to choose to do so . *Triumph over limitation by incorporating flexibility into your thinking.* Reignite the positive flame within you. With enthusiasm, passion, and dedication to being the most excellent you, you can open your mind to the power of positive thoughts, claiming them and believing in them. As for my patients, they routinely focus on saying, "I am loving and positive energy. This energy flows throughout my entire being. My positive energy influences all good things to flow into my life." What type of energies are you attracting to yourself?

The human mind controls destiny and life experiences. Sharpen your thoughts. Think about what life experiences you are living right now. What experiences would you like to see occur for yourself? What goals would you like to achieve today, this week, and this year? There is no time like now to orchestrate the best you. As Dr. Wayne Dyer has stated, "If you change the way you look at things, the things you look at change." You and I hold the power that can bring change in our lives. Realizing it and believing it is not only the key to making changes happen, but it is the gateway to new beginnings. Your beautiful and perfect imprint can be expressed by living your life in relation to what brings you joy and fulfillment; this will result in the expansion of your truest self. All individuals have a silent inner influence, or aura, that is instinctively (unconsciously) present. Have you ever noticed that positive people attract other positive people? When this happens there is a sense of joy. Choose to share positive enthusiasm with others. Your mental attitude powerfully impacts you and influences those around you. Each day is a new beginning. The importance of your happiness matters today. What type of day are you choosing? Positive thoughts bring positive feelings and support emotional well-being. Isn't psychological and intellectual well-being that which we all strive for? We all are born with inner instincts and intuitions. It is when we take the time to truly listen to them that answers occur. Have you ever taken the time to sit back and truly think of the things that make you happy, where your passion lies, the activities you enjoy, and the talents you have been gifted with? Your mental attitude powerfully impacts you and influences those around you. Each day gives us all a chance for a new start. The importance of your happiness matters today. What type of day are you choosing? Isn't it psychological, intellectual, physical, and spiritual wellbeing that we all strive for no matter what our age?

What Ernest Holmes says about age clearly has a positive impact on how we should perceive aging. He says, "Youth is not a time of life—it is a state of mind. Nobody grows old by merely living a number of years. People grow old only by deserting their ideals. Years wrinkle the skin, but to give up enthusiasm wrinkles the soul." Our invisible power, our mind power, is what relates to how we feel about ourselves. When we feel young, no matter what the age, we realize our inner drive can make today count in ways we may not have felt possible. Yet as time passes, this drive seems to fade for many. Thinking in open and unlimited ways is an avenue to creating new dreams or goals.

If you could take a photograph of what your dreams are, what would the picture look like? Would you be happy with the picture or would you like to change it? This is where your imagination allows you to grow and elevate to a plane of unlimited dreams. There are various books written about the power of thoughts and the personal impact they have. As for me, I have embraced the power of thought control. Just as I teach my patients, thought control is there for everyone to use. Practice positive thought control on a daily basis. What positive thoughts excite you? Write them down and read them daily. Believe in them. I recently read something insightful that Dr. McGraw had written: "Your thoughts are behaviors. Choosing thoughts contributes to your experiences, because when you choose your thoughts, you choose consequences that are associated with those thoughts. In addition, when you choose your thoughts, you also choose the physiological events that are associated with them. There is a very powerful connection at work here. Your physiology determines your energy and action level. You are mentally, behaviorally, and physiologically programming yourself to go through life in a particular way." The power of thought should not be taken lightly. Psychological security is available to each and every one of us.

The pattern of conscious thought is dynamic. Each one of you is perfectly designed, born with an inner knowing and the talents, gifts, and human structure specifically created for who you are meant to be. It is important not to judge yourself against others because your dreams and desires are meant for you alone. Each and every one of you has your own imprinted desires and pleasures. Love yourself and let your inner voice lead you to your best blueprint. Don't allow the external world to tell you who you should be. Take control of your thinking and align yourself with the positive gifts of life that the universe offers. You have your own signature style so embrace it sweetly and express who you are joyfully. And always

remember: you are perfectly made, so release your inner strength, energy, and power.

Habits

Forming habits occur whether you are consciously aware of them or not. When you make purposeful choices to form good habits, you are able to create a healthy mind and body. Daily routines vary with individuals, and whether you are mindful of them or not, have significant impact. If something new has recently been incorporated in your daily routine, it is only a matter of time before it occurs automatically. Yet before a habit becomes automatic, we associate cognitive and emotional characteristics with them. Many studies indicate that it varies from 21 days to twelve weeks of consistent behavior to set a habit in motion. What are your daily habits? Journaling your day-to-day routines can provide you with visual awareness of your habits. Start the first journal entry from the time you awaken and finish when you go to sleep. Include the thoughts that start and end your day. As we all know, there are good habits and bad habits that can unconsciously affect us. Be mindful and choose positive thoughts that flow through your thinking. In so doing you can overpower the negative and deliberately promote emotional balance. This will affect all aspects of life, including your decisions and the flow of circumstances that follow.

The human brain is our highly functioning computer for life. Its intricate and complicated design directs all the body's necessary tasks. In addition to regulating these complicated functions, the brain programs new behaviors whether we are aware of them or not. What actually happens when habits are formed throughout our lives? Arrays of studies show that completing the same task over and over again makes it automatic. In 1983, an author named John Bargh defined the term *automaticity*. "'Automaticity' is evidenced by the behavior displaying all or some of the following features-efficiency, lack of awareness, unintentionality, and uncontrollability."

Therefore, it isn't only being consciously in tune with what behaviors and habits fill our day, but whether these habits are causing us harm and imbalance. Each and every one of us should be honest with ourselves in facing these difficult questions. If you and I want to eliminate any bad habit, we have to decide not to do it. It does not matter if it is smoking, overeating, indulging in alcohol, negative self-talk, low self-esteem, or whatever it is we are gripped with. We need to have willpower and allow a higher force or source other than ourselves to lead the way. Additionally, replacing the habit or habits we want to rid ourselves and replace them with positive habits influences life in a good way. Substituting a good habit for a bad habit adds to positive change and helps you become your most excellent. Here is a quote from Aristotle, an ancient Greek philosopher and physician, of whom was very wise. "We are what we repeatedly do. Excellence, then, is not an act, but a habit."

Additionally, positive habits can become the gateway to how you experience life and make a positive impact. Just as daily habitual routines encompass your day, so does your thinking. Do you have habits of positive or negative thinking? Embracing the power of controlled thinking can assist in your personal growth and success. It attracts the flow of positive energy and outcomes. And that which you allow the mind to focus on has the power to carry over to the next day without you even knowing it. Additionally, incorporating habits of daily meditation and positive affirmations is valuable to your routine. If these are new for you, it is important to realize that studies on this subject vary anywhere from 21 days to twelve weeks to form habits; therefore, initiating these positive choices can become invaluable to reaching the most excellent and balanced you. Meditation can be accomplished through listening to positive music, finding quiet moments to focus on thinking a positive mantra, embracing mindfulness, focusing on certain breathing patterns, and setting an intention. The purpose of setting an intention can act as a filter in your mind. By directing thoughts away from the usual ego-driven pathways, an intention towards compassion, for instance, can result in non-judgmental thinking. (www.

reachyogaglenco.com). Lister below are a few examples of breathing techniques to use.

Meditation has been used for hundreds of years and is a powerful avenue not only to bringing positive changes in your life but also to higher thinking. Mindfulness meditation is a western, nonsectarian, research-based form of meditation derived from a twenty-five-hundred-year-old Buddhist practice called Vipassana, or insight meditation. It is a form of meditation designed to develop the skill of paying attention to our inner and outer experiences with acceptance, patience, and compassion. (www.mediationscience. weebly.com for more information.) At the University of California, Los Angeles medical school's psychiatry department, they define this type of mediation as: "Mindfulness is non-judgmental, openhearted, friendly, and inviting whatever arises in awareness. This allows oneself to be open to the inner power within. This can bring balance to your mind, body, and spirit". Explore the different types of meditative music and find one that is right for you.

Every aspect of our lives is interwoven with all the dimensions—the physical, mental, emotional, and spiritual realm. All of these dimensions occur simultaneously, creating who we are. Our bodies are beautifully created masterpieces. Spiritual health is powerful and invisible, that which is always available to us. It is important to respect and honor ourselves and to honor our bodies. Taking proper care of our bodies on a physical level is important not only to our physical health but also to our minds and spirits. It is also important to ensuring that we function with purpose and our highest potential. Purposefully paying attention to the physical state of our health is invaluable to our values and beliefs leading us to becoming our best. The wisdom within all of us can give the gentle direction and insight we need in order to properly care for our bodies. Being mindful and open to our intuitive balance directs us through our life journeys. Essentially, our thoughts have the power to shape us. Guard your thoughts, as they are the gatekeeper to balance and harmony.

Similarly, it is important to realize that taking care of our bodies through exercise, which assists in optimal body development, impacts our spiritual health. Fortitude, willingness, and commitment elevates us to be the best possible. Being strong in body also develops strength in our centeredness as individuals. The outcome of exercising accomplishes more than influencing your body shape; it influences your well-being, state of mind, and sense of self-accomplishment. It essentially impacts the rhythm of mind-body-spirit.

Daily Affirmations

I love myself and am filled with peace and harmony.

I trust myself to make wise decisions with an internal knowing.

Infinite love guides and protects me.

I am living an inspired life.

I believe in myself and am the author of my life.

Meditation

I am abundant and loving energy. My energy is happiness, contentment, peace, and unlimited power. I am boundless light. I am beautifully designed. I am strong and courageous. I am in tune with my inner voice and intuitively led. I am creative and gifted. I am free of boundaries and am living a life full of endless possibilities. I am healthy in mind, body, emotion, and spirit.

Sharpening Your Structure:
The Power of Nutrition

It is health which is real wealth, not pieces of gold or silver. The human body is the universe in miniature. It follows therefore, that if our knowledge of our own body could be perfect we would know the universe.

—Mahatma Gandhi

P roper nutrition plays a key role in maintaining a healthy body. And just as the human body is complex in design and function, so is the biological impact of the foods you and I consume. Balanced and healthy diets support our psychological foundation and structure. In the last several decades, the definition of a healthy diet has been expanded to include the optimization of long-term health (Walter and Stampfer 2014). Have you ever thought about how food choices you make today can influence how you feel tomorrow? Amazingly, our bodies can derive all the energy, structural material, and regulating agents we need from the foods we eat (Whitney and Rolfes 2011). Clearly, our dietary habits and the foods we eat either support good health or invite bad health consequences over time. We as a society are faced with hundreds of nutritional food options, so making nutritional choices that support good health should be everyone's goal.

When you think about the amount of food individuals consume in a day, in a week, or in a month, it can be astonishing. And the type and amount of food we eat in a twenty-four-hour period dictates the number of calories we consume. Nutritional intake is significant in balancing a healthy diet. We are all aware that nutrition is necessary to sustain life, but a vital question to ask yourself is what state of health are you in right now? Are you in a good state of health or in an unhealthy state? Do you have energy, or do you always feel tired? As we all know, the human body comes in various shapes and sizes. Some individuals can be within their normal weight range and not necessarily be healthy. A well balanced diet and active lifestyle support good health and help maintain body weight (Whitney and Rolfes 2011). Food selection is not only central to sustaining our lives but is also interlinked to just how efficiently our bodies work. The chemical breakdown of your food physiologically determines you. When you think about the food choices you have made throughout the years, consider that their chemical components have driven how all your organs, cells, and millions of atoms operate. This is the internal bio-network that determines your building blocks for life.

All individuals have a genetic profile, a blueprint within. And though we understand RNA and DNA, a new field of genetic research continues to expand: epigenetics. This area of study examines how our environment, including the foods we consume, influences gene expression without changing our DNA (Kauwell 2008). Genes control how cells function and when those functions are carried out. (Visit http://ghr.nlm.nih.gov/gov for more information.) Researchers have been studying this for approximately ten years now and have identified that genes have a switch sitting above each cell that can be turned on or off, depending on environmental factors, such as the food we eat. Switching genes on and off can have dramatic consequences for a person's health (Whitney and Rolfes 2011). This gives us a powerful tool to change our physiology. Because it appears that our diets and lifestyles can change the expression of our genes, changing your food selection wisely will assist in improving your health (Nova). Proper nutrition additionally influences how you feel. The nation's health status suffers when adults, young adults, and children eat poorly. It is imperative we all work toward creating a dynamic shift from that of obesity and increased risks of diseases to that of optimal health. Furthermore, this shift needs to occur on a global level in order to have greater impact of improving the health status for all individuals. Improving health transforms lives from limitations to abundance. It is important to understand the truths about specific food choices and just how powerful—negative or positive—their effect is on your internal structural health. Living a healthy and balanced life adds years without inviting the constraints of later-life disabilities. Isn't that what we all want? There are crucial elements of nutritionally optimal health, no matter what the age. One element involves choosing high-quality nutritional foods and beverages rather than those that have sugar and empty fat calories in them. A second element includes exercise and generally how active you are. Both of these elements have tremendous impact on health and assist you in moving forward to be the best you can be.

Wouldn't it be exciting to one day see a significant decline in obesity, in addition to the multiple chronic diseases that occur as a result of obesity? But as for now, the need to fight obesity and sugar addiction is both nationally and internationally pressing. Obesity is a health concern no matter where we live, and it affects young and old alike. Two-thirds of adults in the United States are obese or overweight, and the prevalence of diagnosed diabetes mellitus type 2 continues to increase concurrently with obesity (Whitney & Rolfes 2011). In 2012, more than one third of children and adolescents were overweight or obese (Ogden, Carroll, & Kit, et al, 2014). *Overweight* is defined as having excess body weight for a particular height, whether the weight comes from fat, muscle, bone, water, or a combination of these factors (National Institute of Health, National Lung, and Blood Institute). *Obese* is defined as having excess body fat (*Pediatrics* 2007). Being overweight or obese is the result of a "caloric imbalance," in this case meaning that too few calories are being expended for the amount of calories consumed. Such conditions are affected by various genetic, behavioral, and environmental factors (Office of Surgeon General; Daniels, Arnett, et al.).

As the world we live in continues to change in the arena of agriculture and processed foods, so must our knowledge. Many individuals may not be aware of the significant impact processed foods and sugars have on our health, yet without this important information, we can inadvertently cause poor physiological function. Therefore, elevate your understanding and decrease your poor food choices, as these are essential to having optimal, healthy bodies. For example, are you aware of what sugar consumption does to the body? Over the past several decades, as obesity rates have sharply increased, the consumption of added sugars has reached an all-time high—much of it because high-fructose corn syrup use, especially in beverages, has surged (Malik, Schulze, and Hu 2006). In addition to the sugar in many beverages, high-fructose corn syrup sweetens candies, baked goods, and hundreds of other foods. Furthermore, fructose accounts for about half of the added sugars in the US food supply and 10 percent of the average American's caloric intake (Bantle 2006). There is a continual increase in the sale of beverages filled with fructose even though such drinks are a poor health choice. Have you ever considered what even one sugary beverage does to the human body? One study completed in 2013 showed that people drinking one twelve-ounce sugar-sweetened soda a day increased their risk of developing type 2 diabetes by 18 percent. This study indicates that only a small amount of excess sugar ingestion each day creates havoc in one's body over the long term (EPIC-Inter-Act 2013).

I would like to compare how the body is affected by ingesting sugar over time with what happens if a vehicle is filled with poor-quality or contaminated gas. At first, your vehicle seems to run a little sluggish or inefficiently. After you continue to put the same poor quality gas in your vehicle, eventually it has a hard time running smoothly. Even so, when it unexpectedly stalls or the ignition doesn't turn over, you may seem surprised. Some people may not give much thought to how low-quality gas impedes the vehicle's function, but eventually it results in the vehicle failing to run. Now think about how your body reacts when you ingest moderate to large amounts of sugar over time. After the body is filled with sugar over and over again, the body's metabolism becomes flooded with sugar. This effects thousands of the body's cells. The internal mechanics of the human body slowly and quietly are influenced by this and attempt to control blood sugar levels in the bloodstream, but eventually this becomes ineffective. The once-healthy human engine becomes sluggish and inefficient, and over time the body becomes compromised, gaining weight and becoming resistant to insulin. Eventually, the sugar impedes the internal function of the body and can ultimately lead to system dysfunction.

Now let's take a look at the ingestion of sugar through the lens of medicine. There is an abundance of scientific research that indicates sugar is a dominant link to obesity and disease. And overwhelming evidence shows excess glucose (sugar) to be a leading killer of Americans (*Clinical Journal of Endocrinology Metabolism* 2006). Sugar rewires the brains pathways. Diets full of processed foods and sugar can increase the risk of depression by 58 percent. Sugar inflames the linings of arteries to the heart, increasing the risk of a stroke or heart attack. When sugar bombards the body, skin ages and wrinkles. Sugar overload can damage the kidneys' delicate filtration system. Diabetes is one of the main causes of kidney failure. (Stork, Berman, and Ross 2014).

Interestingly, I recently read an article written by E. Vasques that states, "The public has not yet recognized the magnitude of damage inflicted after consumption of what most consider only a moderate amount of starch or sugar" (2014). Research is conclusive—the longer you wait to tame aged-related blood sugar increases, the greater your odds of succumbing to diabetes and its associated risks of heart attack, stroke, kidney failure, cancer, and blindness. When you pay attention to everything you put in your body, it may be alarming to know how much sugar you are actually consuming. Many experts have brought this to public attention, as it relates not only to individuals here in the United States but also around the globe. Eating too much sugar and empty calories leads to heart disease, diabetes mellitus, lung disease, kidney disease, cancer, and strokes. It is estimated, for example, that more than half of all Americans suffer from one or more chronic disease (Whitney and Rolfes 2011). Yet healthy lifestyle habits, including healthy eating and physical activity, can lower the risk of becoming obese and developing related diseases (Office of the Surgeon General).

Moreover, added sugar is now ubiquitous in processed foods, both as flavor enhancers and as preservatives. The world daily average consumption of sugar and high-fructose corn syrup per person is now seventy grams (or seventeen teaspoons) per day, up 46 percent since thirty years ago, when daily intake was, on average, forty-eight grams. This is the equivalent of 280 calories per day, which is four calories for each gram of sugar (Research Institute, Credit Suisse 2013). Research also indicates that consumption varies considerably from country to country. At the top, the United States, Brazil, Argentina, and Mexico more than double the world average. Some studies find that individuals in the United States actually consume as many as forty teaspoons of sugar a day—Mexico is not far behind, with thirty-five teaspoons per day (Research Institute, Credit Suisse 2013). This being known is important for making good decisions about not only the foods you consume every day but also the beverages. Purposefully choose optimal foods that promote the best health possible for today and for the years ahead. Without a doubt, the goal for all of us is to live healthy lives by avoiding disease conditions.

An article written by Dr. Dwight Lundel in December 2013 holds great importance to us also, as he reveals how processed foods have actually been harming us over the last six decades. He is a heart surgeon who has performed more than five thousand open-heart surgeries, and he shares invaluable information about heart disease and other diseases. His clinical experience in this field gives us strong insight into the harmful effects of processed foods. "Following a low-fat diet used to be the dietary recommendation for avoiding heart disease, as a low fat diet decreases cholesterol levels. Statistics from the American Heart Association show that

75 million Americans currently suffer from heart disease, 20 million have diabetes, and 57 million have prediabetes. These disorders are affecting younger and younger people in greater numbers every year. And experts now argue that sugar intake is the most important cause of what has become a worldwide epidemic of diabetes and obesity". The US Centers for Disease Control and Prevention released a new report in which they indicated that an estimated 42 percent of Americans will be obese by the year 2030. This information is alarming, and it is a wake-up call that good nutritional habits are needed for optimal balance in health.

You and I live in a fast-paced society and have felt the time crunch in trying to accomplish all that each day challenges us to accomplish; so many people have turned to fast food for meal support. The fast food industry has not only expanded our choices over the years but has also created larger sizes to satisfy growing appetites. What were the normal serving sizes of many foods years ago are now super-sized portions. The marketing strategies of many fast food chains have caused people to eat more food, adding unneeded calories. This causes an overload of calories in the body, which eventually can cause weight gain. Digestion and metabolism work diligently in trying to maintain an internal equilibrium of multi-organ functions, but over time, excessive eating taxes the body and causes physiological imbalances. Eventually too many calories eaten day after day results in the accumulation of fat. Weight gain is attributed to hindering the biological balance of the body. Therefore, when it comes to weight management, it is imperative that we as a society take note and make improvements. One way to improve our daily nutrition is to cut down on calories, especially on empty calories that do not have any nutritional benefit to our body. Deleting unnecessary calorie consumption favorably affects our human bodies. Working for years in the medical field has proven to me over and over again that excessive consumption of any food, especially foods high in sugars and empty calories, can cause long-term damage.

Healthy living at any age starts with eating wisely. Significant changes to our eating habits take time and commitment, but the positive results last for years and enhance your life. The journey of weight management starts with first making the decision to transform your health with short-term goals. Having the mindset that short-term goals are the building blocks for success will carry you toward your long-term goals.

Success with Nutrition

It is vital to ask what the best food choices are for your health. Let's take a look at the benefits of eating fruits and vegetables daily and how they supply nutritious elements. Fruits and vegetables come in various colors and textures, which is nature's way of providing us with a variety of healthy nutrients. Incorporating these foods into our daily diet is beneficial to investing in our health bank. There is a great deal to be said for the power of nature. Eating fresh foods is just another way to capture nature, clean and free of processed ingredients. Also consider that a tangerine has approximately fifty calories, a cup of broccoli contains about thirty-one calories, and one cup of potato chips is about 150 calories. Which is the better choice?

There is an array of fruits and vegetables of various colors and tastes. Nature has provided us with some of the most important foods needed for our nutritional well-being. By *clean foods*, I mean they are grown naturally without artificial products. Clean foods, including fruits and vegetables, provide the vitamins, antioxidants, and minerals needed for optimal body function. Some examples of fruits that supply our bodies with vitamin C include kiwis, oranges, watermelon, strawberries, tangerines, grapefruits, and honeydew melons. Vitamin C helps the immune system, heart, and other bodily functions.

Some fruits, such as cantaloupes, nectarines, and grapefruits, provide vitamin A. Many nutritional studies have identified vitamin A as playing a key role in organ function. Other fruits, such as pears, peaches, pineapple, grapes, bananas, and cherries, provide us with potassium. Potassium has a positive influence in our bodies too. It builds proteins and supports muscle growth, in addition to assisting with the electrical flow of energy for our hearts.

Vegetables are another way that nature provides us with healthy food choices that are low in calories. Vegetables have antioxidants and are anti-inflammatory. In addition, they supply us with fiber, minerals, and vitamins. There are a number of vegetables that help maintain nutritional health. Some examples of these include asparagus, broccoli, mushrooms, green beans, cauliflower, and peppers. Scientists continue to conduct studies that indicate just how important eating vegetables and fruits daily are for health prevention and health maintenance.

Dietary Guidelines for Americans, a 2010 publication, also provides important information related to healthy, nutritional eating. These guidelines focus on nutrient-dense foods, such as vegetables, fruits, whole grains, fat-free or low-fat milk and milk products, lean meats and poultry, seafood, eggs, beans and peas, and nuts and seeds that are prepared without added solid fats, sugars, starches, and sodium. These foods combined can provide the full range of essential nutrients and fiber, without excess calories. The oils contained in seafood, nuts and seeds, and vegetable oils also contribute essential nutrients.

Processed Foods and Wheat

As consumers we are bombarded with foods choices filling the shelves in grocery stores. Do you find yourself selecting foods in the produce section or in aisles featuring processed or genetically modified foods? People of many cultures and countries follow improper nutritional patterns of eating. This includes diets high in carbohydrates, sugar, and flour products that can hinder optimal physical and physiological health. Another food choice to take a look at is wheat starches. Wheat starches are complex carbohydrates. *Complex* means that the carbohydrates in wheat are composed of polymers (repeating chains) of simple sugar, glucose. Simple carbohydrates, such as sucrose, are sugar structures with one and two units. An example of this is whole wheat bread. Wheat bread increases blood sugar to a higher level than that of sucrose (*American Journal of Clinical Nutrition* 2007). Wheat products elevate blood sugar levels more than virtually any other carbohydrate from beans to candy bars. This has important implications for body weight, since glucose is unavoidably accompanied by insulin, the hormone that allows entry of glucose into the body's cells, which convert the glucose to fat. Trigger high-blood sugar repeatedly and/or over sustained periods, and more fat accumulation results (Davis 2011). Today, approximately half of all calories consumed by most Americans come from carbohydrates (*Centers for Disease Control* 2010). Therefore, it is important to pay attention to food labels, as many processed foods contain wheat. Some of the most improbable places that you will find wheat are canned "creamed" soups and "healthy" frozen dinners (Davis 2011).

As a health care provider, I believe that health and prevention are essential. All individuals, no matter what age, should have yearly exams in which they are evaluated and assisted in making the changes needed to optimize health. When I see a new patient, I complete a comprehensive health assessment and physical exam. I always ask a variety of questions related to patients' eating patterns, including their specific food and beverage choices. Additionally, I ask about exercise habits, prescribed medications, over-the-counter medications, alcohol consumption, and smoking history. We also conduct lab tests to monitor physiological functions and ensure ongoing internal health. During this time, many patients confess to having a poor diet and to experiencing a variety of symptoms that limit their daily activities.

All patients need to answer questions honestly in order to set specific and attainable self-management goals. Many individuals in various age ranges do not have long-term goals or the proper knowledge to balance their nutrition, complete an exercise regimen, or use the other health tools needed in order to be healthy. These key factors influence life either positively or negatively. Therefore, it is important to make changes. Eat properly and incorporate an exercise plan into your daily life. Importantly, if you make positive changes and remain or become confident in yourself, you will be amazed at all you can accomplish.

As we all know, food affects us physically in terms of weight and physique. Our bodies' compositions reflect our mechanical and physiological health. The goal for all of us should be that of optimal balance so that we can prevent health problems, such as heart disease, diabetes, high cholesterol levels, and others. A healthy body is a key factor to living a dynamic, healthy life.

A second health dimension affected by diet is mental health. The foods we consume are filled with chemicals that cause many chemical reactions to take place in our bodies and are related to our mental health. Have you ever thought about how the nutrition we supply to our bodies affects us on a mental level? Our minds are always responding to the vibrations of foods we consume. Mental balance occurs related to food choices, the time of day we eat, and how much we eat. When we eat too little, our bodies are sluggish. And when we overeat, the body attempts to convert extra calories into working energy with difficulty. It is important not only to be mindful of food choices but to focus on how they affect your mind power. Balanced nutrition assists the brain in functioning with focus, clarity, and energy necessary to perform optimally throughout the day. Similarly, the food choices we make on a daily basis not only influence our mental health and wellbeing but also affect the quality of our lives.

A third and powerful health dimension related to the food we eat is emotional health. Food can have a negative or positive impact on what we experience emotionally. On the positive side, many people relate eating positively to socializing. Some of these social influences include sharing a meal with friends, family, or social events. Doing so gives us the opportunity to connect with one another in conversation and bond, providing us with a sense of belonging and with happiness. Many find enjoyment in planning and sharing in the eating during holidays and special occasions. Emotionally, we may feel fulfilled and satisfied. On the other hand, emotionally, many people can find themselves eating out of boredom or due to feelings of unhappiness, sadness, anxiety, depression, or low self-esteem. Some people fill a void in life by overeating, and in some cases people realize they may have a food addiction. As we all know, some food choices make us feel better than others, which relates to the reward center in the brain. The reward center releases certain chemicals, such as dopamine, which produce feelings of pleasure. An example of this is sugar. It is important to take a look at how food affects your emotions. Though food is needed to sustain the body's energy, it should not control our emotions. If this is occurring, you can, through active and determined decision making, break the invisible hold this addiction has on you. And if food addiction is a personal challenge, treatment is available through counseling and through seeing a dietician.

Furthermore, food and drink choices have a powerful influence on our emotions due to the fact that each food or drink we put in our bodies produces energetic health. Every food or drink has a specific vibration that is created in our body, which fuels how we emotionally feel. The human body functions with energy and vibrations; therefore, the choices we make also affect the energy interwoven with our emotions. Think about the last food or drink you consumed and ask yourself how it affected you emotionally. Emotions have the power to cause cravings of a certain food and can also cause certain chemical reactions related to our emotional selves. It is important to be aware that the quality of foods you and I eat not only determines what nutrients we are placing in our bodies but also fuels the energy we create.

The foods we eat also affect us spiritually, which is the fourth health dimension. Proper nutrition affects our inner harmony and balance. Just as our hearts beat and our lungs breathe in rhythm, the flow and rhythm of the food we eat affects the energy of our spiritual selves. Listening to the inner guidance of the self can assist in transforming your spiritual health and can bring inner peace, harmony, and balance. Eating healthy foods aligns this dimension with your physical, emotional, and mental selves. We are all given this beautifully created and magnificent body that we should respect and care for with wisdom. Being mindful of proper food choices truly has the power to bring all dimensions of our health and lives into alignment.

Daily Affirmations

I am in control of my health and have the willpower to overcome food addictions.

I believe in myself and am in tune with my inner voice.

My mind is free from all negative thoughts of entrapment and limitation.

I am in rhythm with my internal need for proper nutrition.

I love, respect, and honor my body.

Meditation

I am in harmonious balance physically and nutritionally.

I have control over the foods I choose to eat.

Journaling

Taking time to write down your goals is essential. Visualizing your goals has an immense impact on your success. Hold yourself accountable to these goals; suggested goals are listed below. Be determined; your health depends on it.

Week One

Journal all the foods and beverages you consume daily for one week. Include how much water you drink each day, and include the times you eat your meals and the times you eat snacks. Be honest with yourself. At the end of day seven, review the journal and circle the foods and beverages that contain empty calories. Now circle those that have sugar in them.

Week Two

Delete 50 percent of the processed foods you circled from week one, and replace them with fruits and vegetables. Delete 50 percent of the beverages you consumed that had sugar in them, and replace them with non-sugar drinks.

Week Three

Delete the remaining 50 percent of processed foods you circled from week one, and replace them with healthy nutritional choices from previously discussed healthy food groups. Delete all sugar beverages. Challenge yourself to give up sugar for fourteen days.

Week Four

Continue to follow the healthy nutritional plan from week three. Journal the goals you accomplished.

Physical Health: Setting Your Body in Motion

To keep the body in good health is a duty, otherwise we shall not be able to keep our mind strong and clear.

—Buddha

Exercise plays a key role in achieving our best possible health. Exercise additionally decreases stress, improves mood, increases agility and flexibility, improves muscle strength, enhances metabolism, and improves sleep. It improves reflexes, muscle activation, circulation, and oxygenation throughout the body. It furthermore improves bone health by strengthening bone density and decreasing the risk of osteoporosis. Pushing yourself to be routinely active is extremely powerful. Exercise brings benefits to you today and tomorrow and also assists you in expanding the years you can enjoy optimal health as you grow older. Exercise plays a key role in maximizing your physical health. When you take a close look at your state of health, are you active? Physical activity is defined as "any body movement that works muscles and uses more energy than when resting" by the National Heart, Lung, and Blood Institute (NHLBI).

Additionally, when you maximize your physical capabilities, the physical activities you are able to accomplish with exercise, has powerful positive physiological effects with your body. Exercise induces the releases of positive hormones, which are also called *neurotransmitters* (chemical messengers). The neurotransmitters the brain produces include serotonin, dopamine, and norepinephrine. The *International Encyclopedia of Social Sciences* states that when the brain produces serotonin, tension is eased and the subject feels less stressed and more focused and relaxed. Serotonin is what causes our significantly improved moods after cardio training. Furthermore, dopamine and norepinephrine are neurotransmitters that increases alertness in us. Dopamine acts through four major pathways: the mesolimbic (reward and pleasure), mesocortical (cognitive control, motivation, emotion), nigrostrialal (motor control), and tuberoninfundibular (prolactin regulation) pathways. Dopamine is a precursor to norepinephrine and epinephrine, and levels of dopamine are responsive to serotonin. (See www.integrativepsychiatry.net for more information.)

Surge your serotonin by working your muscles. Releasing these neurotransmitters maximizes your most tremendous you. Exercise accomplishes a great deal in our bodies and minds. There is nothing that can replace it. The human body is an intricate design that functions optimally when exercise increases blood flow and improves oxygenation throughout the brain, heart, and all other body parts. When muscles are moving, the human body is at its most efficient. When you really think about it, doesn't setting your body in motion begin with your decision and attitude? If exercise is an area you struggle with, you need a different mindset and self-determination. Achieving and maintaining your best possible health should be a goal you strive for today and for years ahead. The human body is made to move.

When some people hear the word *exercise*, they think it means completing a triathlon or a one-hundred-mile bike ride. But no matter what your goal, striving to be the most excellent you requires some level of exercise. Saying, "I am getting too old to exercise" or "I haven't exercised in years, so why start now?" reveals that your mind is in invisible shackles. I recently read an article about a ninety-five-year-old woman who broke the world record for running in her age bracket a few years ago. She ran a sixty-meter race in 29.86 seconds. Her name is Ida Keeling, and she serves as a role model, as she did not let her age stop her. She was quoted as saying, "Every year I am going to keep doing what I am doing, and when running time comes, if I feel I am ready, I will go at it." This is something she committed herself to doing, and she accomplished it with fortitude. This story is very inspiring, as she did not set limits on herself. She redefined the false notion of her age's limits. Age does not define you or what you can accomplish. She was the ambassador of her capabilities. Are you expanding your physical health or limiting yourself? Redefine your capabilities and challenge yourself.

Working in the medical field, I have the opportunity to care for patients that range from twenty-two to ninety-five years old. Because health and prevention are so important, many patients are now in exercise programs and have amazing health outcomes. I recently took care of a forty-seven-year-old man who was eighty-eight pounds overweight and who was diagnosed with hypertension, diabetes mellitus type 2, and depression. Through an exercise and nutritional program that he committed himself to following, he recently met his goal of losing eighty-eight pounds and has significantly improved his health. He exercises daily and is now off the medication that had been prescribed for him for hypertension, diabetes, and depression. This individual, like many individuals, found that physical activity is an essential component in maximizing health. Clinical evidence shows exercise not only helps prevent type 2 diabetes, but it also lowers blood pressure—and more. New studies show how quality of life, mortality, cardiovascular disease, blood pressure, cholesterol levels, and type 2 diabetes are all affected positively by physical activity (American College of Sports Medicine 2014). As for this particular patient, his journey toward improved health started with him making a personal decision to change his lifestyle. And just like this patient, we all have the ability to change our bodies. It starts with changing our minds. Committing to daily exercise is not only a personal choice but also a commitment to allow this behavioral change to occur. It takes mental resilience to conquer the habit of exercise. Be determined; be strong.

As for myself, I also had to overcome my physical limitations through great adversity after a skiing accident. I had severely injured my right leg, sustaining multiple fractures that required surgery to implant a plate and multiple screws. After months of my fractures not healing, I was unable to walk or perform any of my normal activities. I had been off work for months and incurred many setbacks. At one point, the possibility of amputation was lurking in the dark. This had challenged many aspects of my life, yet I was not going to allow this setback to control my life. It wasn't until five months following my accident that healing started to occur. It took an additional five months for the fractures to fully heal. Yet with many days of frustration and challenges, I did not give up. I was not going to allow this set of circumstances to limit my determination. I worked through days, weeks, and months of intense pain, completing physical therapy daily to regain my physical health. Approximately ten months following my accident, and through many diligent sessions with my physical therapist, I was able to walk again. I had lost a great deal of muscle mass and strength, and it took the next two years of completing daily physical exercise to regain the level of health I'd had previous to my accident. Working with physical therapists had been extremely important. They gave me a plan that they developed to improve my muscle strength and to work all the muscle groups that had been lost with non-use. In looking back at this experience, I can say that I have never taken my physical health for granted. Up to this point in my life I had been able to exercise and do all the activities I enjoyed. Fighting to regain the strength and mobility that which was comprised was worth all the hard work I endured. Moreover, when any type of injury impedes our daily lives, we must look ahead with determination. Physical health is a gift, and we all should take care of it.

Our bodies adapt to all the positive outcomes of exercise. We are perfectly designed. The human body is an amazing machine interwoven and created not only to move but also to recover in extraordinary ways. Your body comes with an internal drive for what you want to accomplish. One of my favorite quotes is by George Lucas, who states powerfully, "Always remember your focus determines your reality." There is a wealth of literature citing clinical evidence that people who consistently exercise have improved physiological functions and lower stress. And since age is a moving target, *today is a great day to exercise*. There are different levels of exercise, from low-intensity to high-intensity, as well as different types of exercises.

What are your goals for physical fitness? Physical fitness is a key part of health. I am a strong advocate for visiting your primary care provider in order to have a thorough physical and health assessment completed. This offers a great deal of important information for you in monitoring your health and assists in setting goals that you can strive to achieve. And remember the benefit of exercise is avoiding the cost of compromised health. Monitoring your blood pressure, heart rate, and body weight are a part of fitness. Many practitioners use the body mass index (BMI) for measuring weight. This calculation is defined as a person's weight in relation to height. Another type of measurement that is used is a person's waist circumference. This is an easy measurement you can do routinely in monitoring your own weight loss or weight gain. A person's waist circumference is a good indicator of fat distribution and central (abdominal) obesity (Depress 2008). As waist circumference increases, disease risks increase (Whitney and Rolfes, 2014). Having a tape measure to see where you are presently with this measurement can influence what goal you want to attain or maintain. A baseline physical assessment includes objective and subjective information that is multifaceted and important to evaluating health risks and health improvements.

The American College of Sports Medicine recommends guidelines for physical fitness that include cardiorespiratory, strength, and flexibility activities. These guidelines recommend the ideal frequency, intensity, and duration of each category of activity.

Cardiorespiratory fitness refers to continuous aerobic activity that uses large muscle groups. The guidelines recommend performing cardiorespiratory exercises five to seven times per week with moderate intensity. This intensity is equivalent to walking at a pace of three to four miles per hour for thirty minutes. Examples include running, cycling, swimming, inline skating, rowing, power walking, cross country skiing, kickboxing, jumping rope, and playing various sports, such as basketball, soccer, racquetball, tennis, and volleyball.

Strength fitness refers to performing resistance activities at a controlled speed and through a full range of motion. The guidelines recommend performing strength exercises two or more nonconsecutive days per week. The intensity is defined as enough to enhance muscle strength and improve body composition. The recommended duration is eight to twelve repetitions of eight to ten different exercises (minimum). Examples include pull-ups, weight lifting, and Pilates.

Flexibility fitness is stretching that uses major muscle groups. The guidelines recommend performing flexibility exercises two to seven days per week. The recommended intensity is defined as enough to develop and maintain a full range of motion. The duration is two to four repetitions of fifteen to thirty seconds per muscle group. An example is yoga. Incorporating stretching and flexibility exercises is important to overall fitness. Moreover, working the center of your body or your torso (core) is essential to physical health. Core strength accomplishes stability, balance and strength in the abdominal and lower back region. Optimizing core strength assists our bodies in multiple body movements.

An important goal in cardiovascular training, if burning fat is one of your goals, is to exert the body sufficiently to burn fat calories. Whenever you choose to exercise in your day, remember that morning cardiovascular training offers the most benefits, as the glycogen stores in the body are at their lowest point in the morning. This, of course, depends on your sleeping pattern; if you're an individual who has a pattern of sleeping at night, then the body will not have consumed food for several hours before exercising, which is ideal. As we know, the body needs energy in order for physical exertion to occur. When the body uses stored fat for this fuel, losing excess weight occurs.

Strength training has a tremendous positive impact on our bodies. Incorporating strength training two to three times per weeks is beneficial to improving strength, flexibility, and bone density, which helps prevent osteoporosis. As for myself, when I think of core strength training, my focus is specific: centered, overcoming, resilient, and exerting (CORE). It is important to be *centered* when performing this type of training. Be aware of your posture and focus on specific muscle groups as they are challenged. The center of these muscle groups is the length of muscles that extends from your neck (cervical) region to the lower spine. *Overcoming* the times when you may not feel like exercising is essential; push yourself to complete your workout and let the desired outcome drive you. Be *resilient*—reaching exercise goals is within all of us, even if we have to dig deep down to finish the workout we planned for a particular day. *Exerting* when we exercise pushes us beyond our comfort zones. When the invisible boundaries of this comfort zone expand, you will tap into an internal self-confidence that you may have never known you had.

An important part of exercising is monitoring your heart rate. The American Heart Association recommends, for most healthy people, an exercise target heart rate ranging from 50 to 75 percent of one's maximum heart rate. Light intensity exercise should result in a heart rate between 50 to 60 percent of one's maximum. Moderate intensity should result in 60 to 70 percent of one's maximum heart rate. Heavy intensity should result in 70 to 85 percent of one's maximum heart rate. The formula for determining your target heart rate is to first subtract your age from 220. This represents your maximum heart rate. Now, multiply that number by the intensity percentage level you have chosen to exercise. (See www. fitnessusa.com for more information.)

According to the Centers for Disease Prevention, a physical activity pyramid they have created indicates the minimum amount of aerobic physical activity people need to engage in, in order to gain substantial health (www. cdc.gov/physicalactivity/everyone) benefits. Therefore, when we think about our individual activity goals, keep in mind that the greater the level of aerobic activities we accomplish, the greater the health dividends we acquire for ourselves. This can be achieved by comparing breathing and/or heart rate, perceived exertion, results of the talk test, energy expenditure, and walking pace. When considering breathing and/or heart rate, note that light intensity will result in little to no increase in breathing or heart rate, moderate intensity will result in some increase, and vigorous intensity will result in a large increase. When considering perceived exertion, use a scale from zero to ten: light intensity will rank less than a five, moderate exertion will rank at a five or a six, and vigorous exertion will rank at a seven or eight. When considering the talk test, note that light intensity will result in being able to sing while exercising, moderate intensity will result in being able to have a conversation but not sing, and vigorous intensity will result in conversation being difficult or broken. When considering energy expenditure, note that light intensity burns less than three and a half calories per minute, moderate intensity burns between three and a half and seven calories per minute, and vigorous exercise burns more than seven calories per minute. Finally, when considering walking pace, note that light intensity means you're walking slower than three miles per hour, moderate intensity means you're walking between three and four and a half miles per hour, and vigorous intensity means you're walking over four and a half miles per hour (www.cdc.gov/physicalactivity/everyone).

Functional training is a type of exercise that assists the body in becoming strong enough to complete daily activities and tasks. As we age, our muscles age also. The activities that were once easy to accomplish can turn into a struggle. When you were younger you might have been able to lift a sixty-pound bag out of the car or climb a flight of stairs carrying two bags of groceries without thinking twice about it, but as we age, these tasks become increasingly challenging until, in most cases, we are unable to do them without help. Functional training provides key stability to our bodies and incorporates muscle groups that focus on specific tasks we do on a daily basis. As we age, we need to keep our bodies active in order to continue to enjoy the things we like to do. Whether you have never exercised or used to and have since stopped, now is the time to motivate yourself to exercise.

Have you ever wondered why you can regain muscle strength fairly quickly when you resume exercising after having stopped for a period of time? Did you know our muscles have memory? Studies have shown the reason why this occurs. Unlike other cells, muscle cells have more than one nucleus (probably thousands). So why do muscles need so many nuclei? The nucleus is basically what controls the cell, and since your muscles are a lot bigger and more complex than other cells in the body, one or two nuclei cannot do the job. So when your muscles get bigger, you have to add more muscle nuclei (See www.exercisebiology.com for more information). There are nearly 650 skeletal muscles in the human body that attach to bones and connect to joints to enable us to move our limbs. There are also muscles that connect muscle to tissue and that connect muscle to muscle (See www. huamn-body-facts.com for more information). When muscles are engaged in exercise, the body is in flow with energy well beyond what we can see.

Therefore, when our bodies are challenged with exercise routinely, our internal blueprints continue to develop. Adding variation to your weekly routine is additionally beneficial. Dr. Adam Knight states, "The more exercises you perform, the more motor units you will recruit, which will activate and build more muscle fibers and reduce the amount of atrophy (muscle deterioration and loss) that comes with aging and inactivity." *The New England Journal of Medicine* revealed that regular exercise can increase a person's expected life span up to almost seven years. Much more important, perhaps, is their finding that exercise greatly increases a person's functional life span. As adults, continued independence is something we all hope to maintain. As time goes on, routine exercise affords us the possibility of continuing to do the things we enjoy doing.

Exercise, in addition to other positive lifestyle habits, significantly impacts all of us. No matter what your age, invest in your "health bank" currently and in the years to come. Why wait? Don't you want this bank account stable? A study reported in the *British Medical Journal* in 2012 concluded that even after age seventy-five, lifestyle behaviors, such as not smoking and engaging in physical activity, are associated with longer survival. A low risk-profile (defined in the study as healthy lifestyle behaviors, participation in at least one leisure activity, and a rich or moderate social network) can add five years to women's lives and six years to men's. These associations, although attenuated, were also present among the oldest (those over eighty-five years old) and in people with chronic conditions. Another study also found that exercise adds years to your life—an additional 12.7 years, in fact, of a healthy, disability-free life. As we grow older, don't we want to live as actively as we can and avoid the limitations or disabilities we could have avoided?

When you think of exercise, do you think about how it affects your brain function? And, just like other muscles in our bodies, if we do not use the brain, it becomes less efficient. When we stimulate the brain through exercise, which can accomplish weigh management, we achieve mental balance. What does exercise do to the brain and to cognition? Increased exertion through exercise increases blood flow and oxygen to the brain, which can produce positive changes at minute physiological levels. The part of the brain most affected by physical activity is the hippocampus. Regular exercise has been shown to counter the shrinking of the hippocampus that naturally occurs in late adulthood. Additionally, through clinical research, Dr. Amen attributes being overweight or obese to decreased brain function in the prefrontal cortex. The prefrontal cortex is responsible for decision making, impulse control, and reasoning. This part of our brain, when in optimal health, assists us in maximizing our thinking and our self- control. The mind is always active, whether at the conscious or subconscious level, so let it guide you with a knowing confidence.

Hydration

What is it that human bodies cannot live without? Water. Water is vital to sustaining our existence. The body instinctively knows how and strives to sustain youthful longevity, but water is key to its process. The human body is over 70 percent water. Our blood is more than 80 percent water, the human brain is over 75 percent water, and the human liver is an amazing 96 percent water. (See www.dorchesterhealth.org/water.htm for more information.) When we think of our bodies functioning and working in perfect sync, we should think of sustaining our magnificent bodies with water. Water has its own energy that physiologically promotes an internal happy world. Have you ever thought of water as simple medicine? Adequate amounts of water daily can prevent headaches, balance body temperature, and promote proper balance of the kidneys, gastrointestinal tract, and blood pressure. Our bodies lose water throughout the day with normal activities. When we increase daily activity with exercise, additional water loss occurs. Therefore, it is important to replace adequate amounts of water daily, in addition to increasing water consumption when you exercise.

When it comes to water replacement, the best way to meet your body's need is to drink water. There is a difference between drinking pure water and beverages that contain water. Fruit juice, soft drinks, coffee, and so on, may contain substances that are not healthy and may actually counter some of water's positive effects. A twelve-ounce can of regular soda contain the equivalent of nine teaspoons of sugar and loads the body with empty calories. (See www.dorchesterhealth.org/water.htm for more information). So when we are thirsty and thinking about what choices we should make, it is recommended to drink water rather than drinks filled with sugar.

Our health's physical, mental, emotional, and spiritual dimensions are interwoven with exercise in powerful ways. Exercise not only involves the muscles and the rest of the body as it moves into a pattern of purposeful activity, but it also is a key ingredient in decreasing stress or other unhappy

42

feelings that influence our physical health. Exercise is empowering and gives us a sense of achievement and pride. This can positively influence how we feel and can invigorate us in all aspects of our lives. As we know, through exercise, powerful chemicals are released in the body and can make us feel happier. Positive emotions bring about a happier heart, and through this energy our spiritual health becomes enlightened.

Daily Affirmations

I am strong and centered. I am positive energy and am in perfect health.

I am confident in who I am and have the willpower to care for my body by exercising.

I illuminate my healthy body through love and kindness.

My time is balanced so that I am accomplishing daily exercise.

I am successful in all aspects of my life.

Journaling

Week One

Journaling your daily activity and exercise pattern is important. If you go walking, write down how many minutes you walked. If you exercise, be specific as to what exercises you completed and how long for each one. (All activities should be included, such as swimming, dancing, bowling, bike riding, running, weight lifting, resistance training, playing basketball, playing tennis, etc.).

Week Two

Journaling what activities or exercises you completed each day and how much time you spent completing each one is helpful to see the progress you make. If no exercising had been completed, start by adding thirty minutes a day three times a week.

Week Three

Journaling how many days you incorporated exercise into your routine last week is helpful in keeping track of your exercise pattern. Increase your exercise activity to four to five times a week, and document how long you engaged in each one.

Week Four

Review the American College of Sports Medicine recommendations discussed earlier in this chapter. The guidelines for physical fitness include cardiorespiratory, strength, and flexibility activities. Use the self-assessment guidelines for monitoring your target heart rate for all activities completed and the level and physical intensity with each exercise.

Eat healthy, live well, and design strong.

References

Agatston, A. 2011. "New Concerns about Gluten." *The South Beach Wake Up Call.*

Bargh, J. 1997. The automaticity of everyday life. In R.S. Wyer, Jr (Ed). The automaticity of everyday life: Advance in social cognition. (Vol.10, pp 1 -61), Mahwah, NJ: Erlbaum.

Brennan, B. 1993. *Light Energy. The Journey of Personal Healing.*

Centers for Disease Control and Prevention. www.cdc/gov/physicalactivity/everyone.

Dudek, S. 2010. "Water and Minerals." In *Nutrition Essentials for Nursing Practice*, 6th edition, 118–147. Philadelphia: Lippincott Williams, & Wilkins.

"EPIC-Inter-Act." 2013.

Holmes, E. 1984. Living the Science of Mind. *Science of Mind Communications.*

International Encyclopedia of Social Science 2007.

Kauwell, G. 2008. "Epigenetics: What It Is and How It Can Affect Dietetics Practice." *Journal of the American Dietetic Association* 108: 1056–1059.

Ludwig, D. 2013. "Examining the health effects of fructose." *JAMA* 310(1): 33–34.

Malik, Schulze, and Hu. 2006. Intake of sugar-sweetened beverages and weight gain; a systematic review. *The American Journal of Clinical Nutrition.* Aug; 84(2):274-88.

Pujalte, G. 2014. *American College of Sports Medicine* 16 (2).

"Position Statement of the American Dietetic Association: Total Diet Approach to Communicating Food and Nutrition Information." 2007. *Journal of the American Dietetic Association* 107: 1224–1234.

Office of the Surgeon General. The Surgeon General's Vision for a Healthy and Fit Nation.

Ogden, C., Carroll, M., Kit, B., & Flegal, K. 2014. *The Journal of American Medical Association.* 311(8):806-814.

Rizzule, D., Orsini, N., and Wang, Q. 2012. "Lifestyle, Social Factors, and Survival after 75: Population Based Study." *BMJ* 345: e5568.

Stork, Travis, Jennifer Berman, and Racheal. 2014. "Your Body on Sugar: An Infographic." *Prevention.*

U.S. Department of Agriculture and U.S. Department of Health and Human Services. 2010.

Dietary Guidelines for Americans, 2010 (7th Ed.) Washington, DC: U.S. Government Printing Office.

Willett, W. and Stampfer, M. 2014. "Foundations of a Healthy Diet." *Modern Nutrition in Health and Disease*, 11th edition, 1455–1469. Philadelphia: Lippincott Williams, & Wilkins.

Whitney, E. and Rolfes, S. 2011. "An Overview of Nutrition." *Understanding Nutrition*. Wadsworth Cengage Learning.

www.definitions.ent/definition/imagination

www.dorchesterhealth.org/water.htm

www.exercisebiology.com

www.fitnessusa.com

www.hsph.harvard.edu/nutritionsource/what-should-you-eat/vegetables-and-fruits

www.huamn-body-facts.com

www.integrativepsychiatry.net/dopamine.html

www.vegan-nutritionista.com/list-of-fruits

www.who.int/mediacentre/factssheets/fs311/en/index.html

www.who.int/mediacentre/factssheets/fs311/en/index.html

www.mediationscience.weebly.com

www.nhlbi.nih.gov/health/dci/Diseases/obe/obe

60101100R00034

Made in the USA
Lexington, KY
26 January 2017